G000130746

Through Your

Doors Again

A journey in poetry from classroom to chemotherapy

Mairead
Best Wishes
Cathy O'Sullivan
24/01/23
xxx

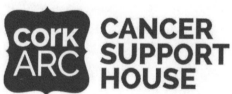

Cathy O'Sullivan
Foreword by Enda Wyley
Illustrated by Rita Dineen

Copyright © Cathy O'Sullivan 2022

978-1-914225-99-4

All intellectual property rights including copyright, design right and publishing rights rest with the author. No part of this book may be copied, reproduced, stored or transmitted in any way including any written, electronic, recording, or photocopying without written permission of the author. Published in Ireland by Orla Kelly Publishing. Cover illustration by Rita Dineen.

Orla Kelly Publishing,
27 Kilbrody,
Mount Oval,
Rochestown,
Cork.

From Classroom to Chemotherapy

You opened your doors to me
when I was eighteen.
I entered as a student nurse.
You were the classroom.

I entered your doors again
on the 16th of March 2021.
This time I was the patient
and you the Infusion Unit.

Acknowledgments

A journey began on 30/01/2021 when I found a lump on my right breast. I immediately made an appointment with my GP and was swiftly referred to Cork University Hospital. My life changed on 22/02/2021 when I was diagnosed with breast cancer. One of my ways of dealing with this diagnosis was through writing poetry, often when sitting waiting for appointments or at moments during the day when inspiration came. The poems are written in date order and are like diary entries to document the various stages of my treatment. This cancer journey is unique to me, as I am aware that everyone's cancer journey is so different. My message to all reading this book is the importance of breast self-check.

There are so many people that I am grateful to for accompanying me on this journey.

Thank you from the bottom of my heart to my husband Kevin and my son John for your unfailing support, patience, and love through my illness and throughout writing this book. I could not have done it without you.

I want to thank Enda Wyley for mentoring me throughout the process of writing this book. Enda's encouragement and superb guidance kept me writing after she read through and edited the first six poems with me. It was easy to write those early poems, but as the time went on my energy and inspiration both fluctuated. One Zoom meeting with Enda and I was reenergised to continue writing. Huge thanks to my niece and Godchild Maria Lynch for her assistance with the final editing and polishing of the poems. Mile buíochas Enda for reading the final manuscript and for writing the foreword.

Thank you to the medical and nursing teams that cared for me at Cork University Hospital (CUH) and the South Infirmary Victoria University Hospital (SIVUH): Professor Seamus O' Reilly (Oncologist), Ms Deirdre O' Hanlon (Consultant), Norma Dowling (Breast care Nurse), and all the wonderful staff in the Orchid Centre in CUH, also the staff in Theatre and in the Glandore Centre in CUH. Thank you to Jackie Depuis (Clinical Nurse Specialist) and all the remarkable team in the Infusion Unit in the South Infirmary. Thanks also to the team in Pathology who did my weekly blood tests prior to chemotherapy. You all do an incredible job with professionalism and kindness.

Thanks to my GPs Dr Jane O' Callaghan and Dr Paddy Hayes of the Fingerpost Surgery and Blackrock Hall. You were always there when I needed you most.

To Fiona and all the team at the Wig Clinic in Barrack St. Cork, and my hairdresser Carmel, your sensitivity and compassion always put me at ease. Thank you.

Thanks to Fiona, June, Hilary, and the amazing team at Cork ARC for your support. I am forever grateful to you all. All monies from the sale of this book will go to Cork ARC.

To Ann: from our student days in the South Infirmary to now you have always been with me…thank you.

Huge thanks and appreciation to my extended family, relatives, neighbours, friends, and my work colleagues at Cork University Maternity Hospital for your continued support during my cancer journey. As there are too many to name and the possibility of leaving someone out, the poem "Gifts" is dedicated to you all. I was deeply moved by the kindness I experienced, and I feel so much gratitude to you all. You will never know how much of a difference you made to my journey. You carried me through it. I will thank you individually when I meet you.

Cathy

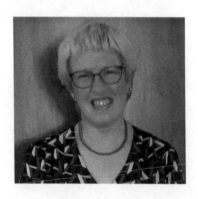

Foreword

The very first poem I read by Cathy O'Sullivan was called 'Swim.' She had submitted it for a poetry workshop that I was running online for the Irish Writer's Centre, Dublin, in October 2020. The poem was one of pure happiness, indicative of the work that I was later to enjoy by Cathy. Written in July 2020 in the early, stressful times of Covid, it described how Cathy and a fellow healthcare worker, found immense relief from the worries of work one July evening by simply going swimming together.

I carried the joy for the night,
and was still bathing in the benefits at first morning light.
All I want to do now is head back to the sea,
and once again feel the joy this experience gives to me.

This exuberance for living, an innate gift that Cathy possesses, was tested to the full when, six months after that joyful swim, in February 2021, she was diagnosed with breast cancer. And yet, just a few short weeks later, Cathy emailed me, wondering did I remember her from the poetry course the previous year, explaining her diagnosis and wondering would I mentor her. She was already receiving chemotherapy every two weeks, she told me, but had written six poems and was hoping to keep writing poetry and to work towards a book about her cancer, the proceeds of which would go to Cork ARC Cancer Support.

Just two months after her life changing news that she had cancer, Cathy began her first poetry mentoring session with me. It is a testimony to her determination, courage and love of poetry that she committed herself to creativity and to seeking out inspiration through her own poetry writing, and that of others, in the sessions that we shared together during this most difficult time of her life. We met on ZOOM every month from April 2021 until December 2021, Cathy's poems inspired by the new, unexpected, challenging time that she found herself in both physically and emotionally.

Now, it is daily appointments
new people, new language.
The whirlwind world of cancer
that I inhabit now
is nowhere I ever thought
I would explore.
'New World'

Sometimes our poetry meetings were delayed or rearranged due to the pressures of Cathy's new life. But Cathy always persisted, ensured that we meet once a month and she never came to any of the sessions without a great sense of purpose and delight in the process of making a poem and discussing poetry with me. It was as though the journey of illness was being eased for her by the new, exciting path that poetry was leading her on. And never one to complain, Cathy always filled the screen of our meetings together with good humour, smiles, laughter and an impressive honesty about her plight.

One of my favourite poets, Czeslaw Milosz, believed that poetry's role was to illuminate the world. Like Milosz, Cathy's poems in this, her debut collection, offer great illumination. They reveal what it is to be ill but also what it is to have hope, believe in life and to recover. To read these poems is to encounter brave work that uncovers what it is to be vulnerable, to feel your life shaken to its very core. But they are also poems that brighten the world with their positivity, insight, wit. Most of all, these poems for all their variety of emotions and thoughts, express what it is to be fully human. Cathy tells it as it is. 'Each challenge provoked/ a new strength in me,' she says in one poem. In fact throughout this collection, Cathy is a courageous poet, who expresses in her trademark natural way, the truth of her experiences.

So now you know it.
I don't have to hide anymore.
I am going through a metamorphosis
and it's full of challenges and occasional bliss.

There is no doubt that poetry has offered Cathy hope and guidance during these challenges. I often turned her attention to reading more poets and learning from their wise and gifted ways. Helen Dunmore, a fine poet, who herself had cancer, offered Cathy enormous inspiration through her poetry. Another poet whose work Cathy encountered during our sessions, was the American Wendell Berry. 'When despair for the world grows in me,' he wrote in his poem, 'In the Peace of Wild Things,' 'I come into the presence of still water./ And I feel above me the day-blind stars/waiting with their light. For a time/ I rest in the grace of the world, and am free.'

It was a joy to enter the pleasurable poems that Cathy wrote during a time of personal turmoil, many of them graced with her sheer happiness at being alive, her sense of what it is to be free. In her poem, 'Response to Diagnosis,' she freewheels down a hill in Cork city and we feel as readers, an overpowering sense of relief, feel as exuberant as the poet herself.

> *This is nothing like freewheeling*
> *down Donnybrook hill soaking*
> *in the beauty of the city spread*
> *out in front on a sunny morning.*

Gratitude also plays an enormous part in Cathy's poetry. In her poem, 'Gifts,' she is grateful for the kindness of neighbours, family and friends, who helped in so many ways but most importantly, 'Let me talk, allowed me to be silent./ You listened and really heard/even when I did not utter a word.'

Throughout these poems, Cathy celebrates each moment of being alive, often with a poignant humour. In the poem, 'Dog days,' she is suffering the 'new indignity,' of having her hair shaved at home in her kitchen but finds solidarity in the form of her husband's and son's unexpected and loving action.

> *Surprise took over as I noticed*
> *my son's shaved head and my*
> *husband's skint-tight haircut.*
> *All of us bald together.*

Mary Oliver in her poem, 'I Worried,' finally gives up worrying, sees that it came to nothing, and 'took my old body/and went out into the morning,/ and sang.' Like Oliver, Cathy O'Sullivan's poems are the music of her own life's new song. They are the songs of how she feels and thinks during cancer, the challenges she faces, the people who she loves and who have loved her back. They are songs too borne out of the comfort of nature and the sea and of her yearning to celebrate the world she is very much present in, very much a part of. I feel truly blessed and so privileged to have been taken on this journey by Cathy through her wonderful poems. May the muse always be with her and may her poems flow on!

Enda Wyley, Poet, Dublin, March 2022

Enda Wyley has published six collections of poetry, most recently, *The Painter on his Bike,* Dedalus Press, 2019. She lives in Dublin and is a member of Aosdána, the affiliation of Irish artists.

Contents

For
Kevin, John, Liz, John, Maria, and Mary.

Breast clinic (visit 1)

Sitting.
Going nowhere.
Pencil scratching across envelope,
etching away at my disbelief.
My sisters are awaiting
their own fate too.
It is everywhere,
the fear that engulfs our thoughts
and clouds our minds.
It is visible in the eyes,
impossible to disguise,
but deep underneath is untapped
courage that will see everyone through
this journey, this unexpected roadmap.

Behind are families, spouses,
children, siblings…
unexpectedly dragged without
choice on this unchartered journey
carrying their own fears and worries.
Did not ask for the road with the twists and turns,
no turning back, only one way through.
This could happen to anyone, even you.

11/02/2021

Breast clinic visit 2: Diagnosis

I stare down from the ceiling
at the doctor explaining to the woman
on the chair who looks like me
"You have cancer in your right breast"
My eyes are dim and cannot really
focus on the Tsunami that has
invaded the quiet consulting room.

Luckily, the nurse is writing notes,
as I ask each question three times
and still cannot comprehend the answers,
or absorb words:
chemotherapy, surgery,
Oncologist.

22/02/2021

Response to diagnosis

This is nothing like freewheeling
down Donnybrook hill soaking
in the beauty of the city spread
out in front on a sunny morning.

For fear can swallow you
and leave all reason
outside of your grasp
when you need it most.
Trust is a big ask
in the deep end
of the unknown.

22/02/2021

Waking up to reality

All week I have not been able to sleep
Lying awake in the dark
dealing with my darker thoughts.
My unfocused gaze fixed
on the dim glow of the calving monitor.
Observing the cow giving birth,
I deeply desire some of her calm.
I had got some news
that started to melt
my plans for the future
and my sense of self.

Nobody expects it to be them
This always happens to somebody else
Now '*I realise that somebody else
is actually me*'.

27/02/2021

New World

Traumatic shock
force of lightning
unsteadies me
knocks me off my pedestal.
I shatter into a thousand pieces,
as I try to piece together
this new world I find myself in.

A moment mid-flight
from Rome to Bangkok
in 1982 to the refugee camps
along the Thai border
I knew there
was no turning back.

Now, it is daily appointments
new people, new language.
The whirlwind world of cancer
that I inhabit now
is nowhere I ever thought
I would explore.

11/03/2021

Egghead

No words today.
What can I say?
My hair will all
fall away.

Egghead, I think.
No more leaning
over the sink, no more
shampoo in my eyes.

It grew up with me –
through the toddler years,
the teen years, into adulthood,
through the decades.

No words today.
What can I say?
My hair will
all fall away.

But go it must.
Onto the pillow, into the bin.
I will be as bald
as a baby once again.

12/03/2021

(For Carmel, my friend and long-time hairdresser, and my cousin Rosarie who introduced me to zany hairstyles when I was a teenager.)

Rat Night

Rat night –
more like a cat fight,
I thrashed and turned,
shivered and worried.

As the DTs ripped my body
I felt lost and shoddy,
wanted to flee from it all –
my time of derogation.

Good cells, bad cells.
What the hell!
An internal inferno –
no place of comfort to go.

Hell hath no fury
Like bad cells scorned.
Chemotherapy is rough
Please be warned!

To the core, to get the strength
to fight this –
as each bad cell goes through
its chemotherapy kill.

In the midst of my life's worst
scare. In the midst of Covid
I could have been alone.
But I was cocooned at home.

21/03/2021

(For Kevin and John)

Impact

Losing my hair,
the pain took by shock.
It reminded me I was alive
just about!

It reminded me of the birth
of the placenta, where pain
took me by surprise.
I thought I had it all done
by giving birth to my son.
But there was more to come.

04/04//2021

Dog days

As you shaved my head
I sank further into the chair
in the kitchen and succumbed
to this new indignity.

I looked out the window
and noticed that Tiny and Skype
were simultaneously being trimmed.
I stepped outside to admire their
new look and patted them silently.

I walked out the lane
feeling sorry for myself.
Eventually, I came back home,
I could have bawled.

Surprise took over as I noticed
my son's shaved head and my
husband's skint-tight haircut.
All of us **bald** together.

05/04/2021

(*In memory of Skype*)

Rocky terrain

Bone pain, nerve pain-
This is all new terrain
in the world I have entered
since my cancer diagnosis.

I never knew these effects existed
I was oblivious to it all,
as the drugs do their healing
unquietly.

I sometimes feel like a ferocious
storm is happening inside me.
The journey is rocky
the scenery outside is blurred.

I have to remind myself to breathe
and believe I can get through this.
As a woman journeys through labour
knowing it will all be worth it in the end.

08/04/2021

No one can burn a saucepan quite like my son

You put the batch cook meal together
I handed over the reins
You put in all the ingredients
The recipe is yours now.

The saucepan got a shock.
It had never before gotten such a warm bottom.
You stirred now and again
Some things did not quite blend in.

They stuck to the saucepan floor
Never to be recognised any more
Somehow it all came together.
And you had food for the week.

John, John, what have you done?
Said my lovely saucepan about its bum.
Black and red and sore
Ne'er to be fully cleaned any more.

11/04/2021

Telling it as it is

I want to share my news.
I want to get it out.
My breast cancer diagnosis
Is what this poem is about.

I wear a hat on my head.
It sits where my hair once grew.
I got lots of colours to choose from.
I hope you like today's one!

The past few weeks have been strange
with lots of new experiences.
Each challenge provoked
a new strength in me.

So now you know it.
I don't have to hide anymore.
I am going through a metamorphosis
and it's full of challenges and occasional bliss.

The kindness of family, neighbours, and friends
is the blessed catalyst that gets me through the daily grinds.
So, thanks to everyone for journeying along
as I write the music to my life's new song.

17/04/2021

Gifts

You dropped in dinners.
Did my weekly shopping.
Shaved my hair.
Dried my tears.
Kept me in your prayers.
Accompanied me on short walks.
Sent me cards, flowers, books.
Regular texts, phone calls
Gifts, gifts, gifts…
Updated me with news
and didn't expect a response.
Let me talk, allowed me to be silent.
You listened and really heard
even when I did not utter a word.

06/05/2021

Sea Balm

Fine weather, and a need for solace
steer me in the direction of the sea.
Traces of childhood
linger in the sand.
Waves lapping on the shore fill
me with unexpected energy.

On the horizon lays Ballycotton Island.
I swam towards in my youth.
This beacon of freedom
now lends me strength.

17/05/2021

Hovering

Between letting go of a rollercoaster,
and plunging into a landmine,
between food aversion and food obsession,
and the need for maintenance and building of muscle mass,
I think of Val's words in the toddler parenting class,
"Be a thermostat not a thermometer"
Swinging between internal reactions
I wish I could soothe my body's tantrums.

11/05/2021

https://www.daveynutrition.com/

https://www.valmullally.com/

Winter Retreat

(On your marks, get set, rest…)

My brain is changing,
or perhaps just rearranging
how I think and write poetry.
Perhaps like the seasons,
It needs a rest.

Sleep, creativity, sleep.
It's ok to take a rest.
Like the hibernating animal
you will awake fully refreshed,
in your own time.

14/05/2021

Refuelling

A breath is taken in,
stress is breathed out,
and peace settles in its place.
Like an aeroplane stops to refuel
midway on a long-distance flight.
So, I am replenished when
close to the sea at Myrtleville.

17/05/2021

What anybody else thinks of me is none of my business

I'm precious about my hands.
I want to preserve the veins there.
I want to be able to drive,
and have some element of freedom.

I cry easily and cannot hide my distress.
I'm sorry you are the one to have to deal with this.
It is my world, my reality.
I must stop worrying about what you think.

From the midwife/nurse and teacher
to becoming the patient has overthrown me.
Years of being a carer and trying to empathise
I can't help now but see through the nurse's eyes.

From wellness to illness is challenging.
It is a change no one wants to encounter.
Like the veins in my hands that have endured
and accepted the insertion of all the needles,
I too reach a place of acceptance.

19/05/2021

Uncertainty

I have experienced it before. It has come
knocking at my door. I mustn't rush
my thoughts through to the end. I need
to embrace uncertainty as my friend.

Uncertainty leads to a future unknown.
A time of being fully in the present.
Sometimes immobilised, rooted to the spot.
To experience the absolute now.

To feel whatever it is that I feel.
To think whatever I think.
To live without a plan.
One moment at a time.

21/05/2021

Oblivion

I open the book.
I fall into its pages
and delve into the story
of someone else's life.

It takes me away from mine
and gives me joy.
Trying to knit together,
the characters in the story.

As their lives unravel
and their stories become more complex.
As the mystery unfolds.
I become engulfed in another world.

As the tourist meets the native on the island
and knows nothing of their past.
Then willingly enters a fishing boat.
Who knows where it will take us?

For while I am in the realm of the book.
I can safely enjoy solitude,
and let my mind feed
on the work of another's pen.

It reminds me of diving off the pier
at Knockadoon, when I was sixteen.

Learning to life save in the midst
of fishing boats, the sound of seagulls
and the smell of seaweed in icy cold
water in the middle of summer.

Now books are my life saviour

23/05/2021

What we cannot have is what we most want

All along I dreaded chemotherapy on a Tuesday. I dreaded the needles, the side effects, the symptoms, and the indignity of the cancer.
Today, as I wait anxiously for my blood results which are delayed due to the Cyber-attack, I wish I was in the chair in the Infusion Unit getting the chemotherapy that I previously dreaded.

25/5/2021

Responding to Chemotherapy

You heal me,
and you scare me.
The weekly infusions,
the dreaded needles.

The unyielding veins
that are now so tired
from being pierced each week
blood out and drugs in.

Yet, it is part of a process.
Like a field being ploughed.
To prepare for new growth.
New beginnings.

25/05/2021

Thankful

I'm thankful for the medics.
Helping me to piece together
the elements of my new existence.
Guiding conversations about
topics that I could not start…

I look with awe at your professionalism
and absorb each word with intensity.
I observe your actions, your note taking,
your comforting smile
and offer my heartfelt thank you.

29/05/2021

Thanks to the dishwasher

Thanks for cleaning the ware.
Thanks for doing a chore that I hate.
You continually clean the cups, plates,
cutlery and saucepans.
How come you never get bored?

06/06/2021

Holding my breath

From initial diagnosis
to this present moment
past the halfway mark
I feel like I am holding
my breath, waiting…

Exhale, exhale.
Let it all go.
This too will pass.

10/06/2021

Projects/Adventure

You took on curtains, I took on poetry.
Each of our projects carried us through
the ocean of unexpected illness,
to draw creativity from our core.
Like toddlers draw and create art,
willing to experiment with new colours and shapes,
we eagerly watched our landscape
unfold over the weeks and months
that eventually brought us our finished creations.
You hung your curtains; I published my poetry.

14/06/2021

Recalibrating

It was new and I had to find a way
to adjust to this different situation.
As a toddler learning to walk,
a parent adapting to life without sleep,
these helped me believe I could navigate this.

Halfway through the chemotherapy journey
that road is familiar now.
What was unknown and daunting
is now my new normal.

21/06/2021

The things I have taken for granted

Hair that grew naturally on my head,
Eyebrows that adorned my eyes.
A nose that is not blocked, bleeding or running every day.
Taste buds that identified individual flavours,
No metallic taste in my mouth.
A calm gastrointestinal tract.
Healthy fingernails and toenails,
Sensation in my fingertips,
The ability to open bags and tins.
Clear skin free from rashes.
Weeks free of appointments,
days free from side effects.
Unbounding energy,
an ability to stay awake for a full day.
Being able to go for walks
without having to stop to catch my breath.

04/07/2021

No man's land

In between yesterday and tomorrow
I deal with my new reality.
Like a trapeze artist mid-air.
Swinging, turning like the wheels
of a train on a runaway track.
Onwards I hurtle.

29/07/2021

Birdsong

I'm out in the field bringing in the cows
serenaded by birdsong floating from the trees.
Glorious as the dawn chorus that wakes me
at five am, the sweet sound of daybreak.

The dogs bark in their excitement
scampering along beside me,
making our way to the hum
of the milking machine.

04/08/2021

It is this moment

Awakening to the next chapter,
I leave behind the last difficult
few months and put on wings
to glide into the next phase of this journey.
I try to find a seat belt and a safety net,
they haven't emerged just yet!
I tell myself *"Breathe"*

05/08/2021

Surrender

As I wait to be called for surgery, the busyness
of the admission ward reminds me of
the London underground at morning rush hour.

I think of Helen Dunmore and how she was so calm
to notice a waterfall and compose a poem about it
while the anaesthetist was counting backwards.

As I sit waiting, I'm in the nurse's shoes in my mind
planning and organizing my day, flying around
making sure everything is in order.

But it's not, I am the patient.
How could I be in charge?

06/09/2021

Post-Surgery Lull

They told me to do
nothing. As I watch the loads
of washing mount up and the dust
settle on the windowsill, I fret …
and then connect to my breath.

Still. Be still, I tell myself,
as angels drop in food
and stop to say hello –
these days that are
blessed with healing.

11/09/2021

My love of the sea

The sea is a tonic,
it sustains me.
The ebb and flow.
Always there in the past,
always there for evermore.

I treasure the gift of the sea.
Growing up I cycled there every day.
Like a message in a bottle
I left my cares and worries
float away.

17/09/2021

Affirmations

The food
of my soul –
make me feel
positive
and whole.

I will do them
each day
to keep me
optimistic
all the way.

17/10/2021

Sunday musings

How do I nudge myself
to take up the pen
and make my writing
come alive?

Procrastination, the thief of time,
or friend to pace myself?
Tiredness pulled me back,
sucked away my energy.

I wrestle with my pen,
and write one word again.

26/10/2021

Tearful day

If my tears could talk,
what would they say?
"Go look after yourself,
stop worrying about
housework today"

If I listened to my tears
What would I do?
I would go for a walk
and listen to nature too.

If nature could talk
What would she say?
"Go and take care.
There is nothing more
healing than fresh air"

If I listened to nature
What would I do?
I would throw on thick stockings
and put one foot into each shoe.

I would walk and listen
and see the leaves glisten
in the autumn air -
I would let go of every care.

So, thank you nature for being my friend
and accompanying me on every road and bend.
You are always there, fresh and clean.
In each field, tree and running stream.

20th Oct 2021

Woman in cafe

Latte arrives.
Dream stuff.
In her mind she is
in Italy now.

First sip, liquid gold.
Cancer doesn't belong
in this world.
In this moment.

Yet, it resides her body.

It has no discretion
no class distinction.
It arrives, uninvited-
takes up residence
and pays no rent.

22/10/2021

Next chapter

Turn the page you are stuck on.
Live life to the full and have
some fun. Grab a pen and write
a note, it could be the start
of a great book.

Life – it always blows towards
us the seed of the next crop.
Cultivate from within.
Go forward…
and simply dance and sing
and live on a prayer and a wing.

28/10/2021

Staring at the ceiling

Where else would you see
trees on a ceiling?

Is it lying on the floor
of a polytunnel?

No, it's my current view
lying here- first
dose of radiotherapy.

04/11/2021

Storm Barra

The tall red flowers bend
with the force of the wind
and regain their composure
before the next gust arrives.

07/12/2021

Cork ARC Cancer Support

With Cork ARC
you are never alone.
When you have a concern
pick up the phone.

It takes courage, it takes strength.
But ARC will cushion a world
in which cancer has invaded
your life and your equilibrium.

A listening ear, a soothing voice,
practical support, therapies,
exercise, information seminars.
A plethora of choices.

No charge, no judgement.
Anything that can surface
will get an empathetic response.

A cushion of calm.
It is your space.
Your safety net.

12/1/2022

www.corkcancersupport.ie

About Cork ARC

Dear Reader,

Cork ARC is a safe haven for people with cancer and their families, where you can find information, practical help and emotional support. Whatever stage of your cancer journey, you are not alone. If you are a cancer patient or someone close to you has cancer, they are there to offer you specialist professional support.

All proceeds from the sale of this book will go towards covering the costs of providing services and support at ARC House in Cork City and County, Ireland who do incredible work in supporting anyone going through cancer. Your purchase of this book will help them to continue their vital work. Please also share the word about this book so more funds can be raised. To find out more about Cork ARC go to corkcancersupport.ie. Cork ARC have provided and given permission to use their logo on this book. A copy of the permission can be viewed by mailing the author on cosullivan23@gmail.com.

Thank you for your support.

Cathy

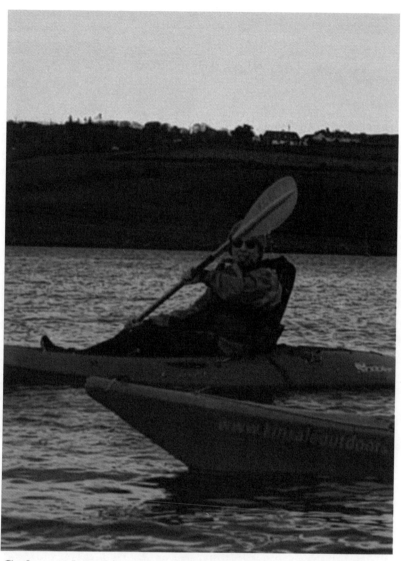

Cathy out kayaking with the 'Ladies who Launch' group in Kinsale, kindly supported by Cork ARC, Canoeing Ireland, Kinsale Outdoor Education Centre and Amy Walsh, Chartered Physiotherapist, Max Physio in Clonakilty.

Resources

Enda Wyley (2019) *The Painter on his Bike,* Dedalus Press,. Dublin.
https://booksforbreakfast.buzzsprout.com/

Helen Dunmore. (2017) *Inside The Wave*. Bloodaxe Books. Northumberland.

https://corkcancersupport.ie/

https://www2.hse.ie/wellbeing/how-to-check-your-breasts.html

https://www.mariekeating.ie/

https://www.daveynutrition.com/

https://www.valmullally.com/

https://www.breakthroughcancerresearch.ie/

https://irishwriterscentre.ie/

Wig clinic. 133 Barrack St, Cork.